MW01182003

CHANGING LIVES ONE SMILE AT A TIME

THE STORY OF DR. HOOKOM'S PERSONAL ADVENTURE AND HOW HE HAS TRANSFORMED LIVES ALONG THE WAY

Published by CelebrityPress®, Orlando, FL.

CelebrityPress® is a registered trademark.

Printed in the United States of America.

ISBN: 978-0-9975366-7-6
LCCN: 2016953583

Most CelebrityPress® titles are available at special quantity discounts for bulk purchases for sales promotions, premiums, fundraising, and educational use. Special versions or book excerpts can also be created to fit specific needs.

For more information, please write:
CelebrityPress®
520 N. Orlando Ave, #2
Winter Park, FL 32789
or call 1.877.261.4930

Visit us online at: www.CelebrityPressPublishing.com

CHANGING LIVES ONE SMILE AT A TIME

THE STORY OF DR. HOOKOM'S PERSONAL ADVENTURE AND HOW HE HAS TRANSFORMED LIVES ALONG THE WAY

By Dr. MATHEW HOOKOM, D.D.S.

Owner of Custom Dental

CelebrityPress®
Winter Park, Florida

Disclaimer

The information shared in this book is intended to provide information that is deemed important to consider when determining if dental implants are a good choice for you. It is not meant to be a substitute for actual consultation or for more thorough evaluation with a professional to determine a properly defined course of action for you.

CONTENTS

CHAPTER 1

THE REWARD OF MY JOURNEY

You are never fully dressed without a smile.
~ Song from the Broadway musical, *Annie*

Providing people with a service that lasts forever and substantially improves their lives and even their health is so exciting for me. The journey to get to this amazing career that I have today in Atoka, Oklahoma and its surrounding communities has been fun and interesting, and there are no doubts that I am exactly where I was meant to be.

When I was younger, if someone would have said to me, "Matt, you're going to be a dentist some day and find that you're passionate about dental implants," I would have laughed it off and thought they were way off base. Me? No way. My family was a hard working family who instilled a great work ethic into me, but it was not a college-bound family. In fact, I was going to be the first one to go to college, but my dreams were not aligned with becoming a dentist. I was the hard working and stubborn guy from Guthrie, Oklahoma. No need to over-think things too much.

Somehow, despite myself, by the good grace and love of God, things did fall into place. Dentistry was part of it and the other part, just like in so many stories, started with a girl.

I have always been able to see God's plan on my life. That plan led me to sit next to a kid on a train in the sixth grade. This kid's name was Nate Brown. Tragically, Nate had lost his brother at a young age to a drowning accident, so what started out as us being best friends, ended up being a situation in which we became more like brothers. His dad happened to be a dentist and was a father-like figure to me. Where my father had instilled hard work and some may say a bit of stubbornness in me, my best friend's dad, Dr. Kelly Brown, taught me about the world of business that he understood so well. Through him I learned lessons on running a business, how to manage money, and also a ton about entrepreneurship. Within the lessons of entrepreneurship, I saw something that appealed greatly to me and how I wanted to live my life:

With the best use of my gifts and talents, I could change others' lives.

God gave me many talents and created me to serve others, He had a plan that was being revealed to me more and more. I listened to a lot of great leaders like John Maxwell, Craig Groeschel, and Andy Stanley, and through their leadership teachings I was inspired to grow spiritually and in leadership. I wanted my life to be better and make others' lives better; by the time college came I had a vision and I was set to go.

My best friend had gotten into college on a golf scholarship and I had decided to attend the same university—East Central University. Since I'd played high school basketball, I decided to check out the college team and see if I could play there. I went and asked about it my first day, and I ended up getting a college scholarship to play. That lead to four years of basketball and scholarships every year thereafter.

I started my college career majoring in pre-engineering. Things were really on track, but I quickly learned that I wasn't really meant to be an engineer, despite loving to focus on specific little nuances of a project and find solutions. So my pursuit of "the right major" continued on. I went to physics, then to computer science, and then to wildlife biology. Quite a diverse range of majors, but many times in college, you really do not know until you've tried. Then, one of my biology teachers, Dr. Choate, said something to me based on his knowing that I was an on-the-go and fast-paced person. He said, "I know you love being outdoors, hunting and fishing and all, but you do realize that you're more likely to be counting snails on a tree than doing anything with hunting and fishing with this major, right?" Umm...what!

At the time I became aware of that, Nate had decided to go to dental school and prepare himself to follow in his father's footsteps. He suggested that I might try it, but I was not ready for a career like that. Me, a dentist, it didn't really make sense. I was insecure about it and I pushed it aside, despite his encouragement and even the encouragement of a few of my teachers. As we all know, when we don't recognize our potential others can talk about as much as they want, but it's not likely to work. But eventually, I did decide to go to school for a dental hygiene degree. And I did right after I graduated from college.

At East Central I became good friends with one my basketball teammates named Ryan. We had a lot in common, including hunting and fishing. He would invite me to his family's land in Atoka for weekends to hang out at his family's house and hunt. His entire family knew me and I knew all of them, except for his sister, who was in college—I'd only met her once, briefly. She was really beautiful, but my friend's little sister. "Stay away" warning signs flashed through my mind. But really, I was busy and life was good.

As time went on, I continued working hard to earn my dental hygiene degree and I had finally stopped being so stubborn and unsure of myself and recognized something that changed my life: I could be a dentist and I did want to be a dentist. Yes, I'd found my why!

I began to work harder and study harder, eager to make it my reality. Wonderful things started to happen that transformed me into a more mature and prepared person. I had learned how to study better and further developed my leadership skills. I saw these things as essential parts of achieving my goal of becoming a dentist. The schooling is strenuous and the expectations are high—as they should be.

Then I got the call. "Hi, Matt, this is Emily, Ryan's sister. Can I ask you a few questions about becoming a dental hygienist? I'm interested in that field." *Of course*, I thought. Well, I must have offered quite a passionate case, because six months later she was in dental hygiene school and my fiancé. In 2007, we were married.

So much was happening and life in the real world was great, constantly on the go. But the more I learned, the more energy and passion I had for dentistry. I'd even set up a plan to partner with Dr. Kelly Brown with the office he was going to open up in Kingfisher. However, with my marriage to Emily, the plan changed. We ended up in Atoka, deciding that was where we would begin our life together.

My mentor, Dr. Brown, had a friend who wanted to start their own practice, but they needed some help. At first they thought why not join forces and become associates, but they both knew that the chances of that being successful was slimmer than either cared for. However, the entrepreneur mindset of my mentor came out of him, and he thought, *what if I could take my 30+ years of experience and knowledge and help other dentists reproduce the culture and systems that I have in my office?* Then he did.

Today, my mentor's vision is what is known as Custom Dental, and it has become my home away from home. I own my own Custom Dental in the town that I first saw my future wife. I actually live in the same house where I first met her, hunt the same land that I loved to hunt in college with her brother, and everything has come together perfectly. God has lead me with His Grace to this exact place to do His work and serve Him... it is just funny when you look at all the pieces that have made up this puzzle called "my life."

I have everything to smile about, which is why I am so vested in helping others smile too.

Early on, I saw the benefits that dental implants offered people and how they could change people's lives. I wanted to focus my learning on implants, but ran into a problem. Since the technology was so new, my school did not teach on implants. So, despite a full school schedule, I began taking weekend courses on everything implants. By the time I graduated, I was able to transform people's smiles with implants. Just thinking about the plights of people who have dentures and how problematic they can be inspires me. People should have complete freedom to enjoy their lives without having to worry about dentures falling out, having to always have a carrying case or denture adhesives on hand. Yes, the powders and creams do help, but just for a few hours. I just didn't think that anyone should have to live that way, and with dental implants, they would not have to!

Sure, there were other options, such as bridges, but even they are not a permanent solution. There is no other long term solution other than dental implants. And they do more than bring back your teeth, they also bring back your smile, improve your health, and help you to do all the things that a life well lived includes— dining with friends, smiling with loved ones, and having the confidence to look the world in the eye.

Every year, I continue to take extensive continuing education and training on everything related to dental implants and other techniques that help people have a better experience with their visit to the dentist. I want them to walk through those doors knowing that without a doubt, and through my team and our actions, we care about their lives and their results. It's not just words, it's what we do.

Dental implants are a standard of care and the best thing in dentistry.

It might seem strange to hear a guy share information so animatedly and with such excitement about dental implants, but if you're reading this book there's a good chance that you are thinking they are an option you need in your life, for some reason, and you understand the association with the challenges of bad or failing teeth, poor dentures, or other dental solutions that just do not work well for a long time, if ever. Knowing that I'm someone who can help you inspires me no end. When people share their experiences at Custom Dental with my staff and I, we know we've come across something special. People like J. Harittag from Atoka write: *I have had several dental issues taken care of by Dr. Hookom and his team. I am very pleased with everything. I used to hate the dentist's office, but now it doesn't bother me as much! Thanks Dr. Hookom and your team for the excellent service and work you provide.* And this is just one example of hundreds of reviews that are available online and throughout the community and surrounding areas our practice serves.

In the end, all I really know for sure is that God blesses us with a lot of talents and he tries to connect us with them. My team and I do what we can for Him and are filled up by the joy of servitude to people in need in our community. Whether someone needs a hug, a full mouth reconstruction, a smile, or just an encouraging word—it's all part of what we do. It does not matter, as we give freely and without expectation.

> *I have found a dentist who I can trust to treat me with care and honesty. The staff treated me with such kindness, and it made the dental work a pleasant experience. I was completely satisfied, and Dr. Hookom followed up with a phone call that evening to make sure I was feeling okay.* ~ Yvonne Walker, Antlers

People want to be healthier and feel good about themselves in the world. I truly believe that and I see it every day through the interactions I have with patients. Dental implants are not just cosmetic in nature, they are essential in nature for many people, and in this book, you'll learn why. They are not for a certain age group, either. People of all ages need dental implants and everyone should experience the dignity of having confidence to look anyone in the eye and talk without worrying about someone focusing in on their mouth instead of their words. And those beautiful smiles...well, we all have one and just like every time a bell rings an angel gets its wings, every time we smile we are giving ourselves and the recipient a gift from the heart.

CHAPTER 2

DENTAL IMPLANTS: WHO WANTS THEM AND WHY

I love smiles. That is a fact. How to develop smiles? There are a variety of smiles. Some smiles are sarcastic. Some smiles are artificial-diplomatic smiles. These smiles do not produce satisfaction, but rather fear or suspicion. But a genuine smile gives us hope, freshness. If we want a genuine smile, then first we must produce the basis for a smile to come.
~ Dalai Lama

Since 2009, I have witnessed some of the most touching stories about people who were desperate for a solution with their teeth. Situations can happen where people lose teeth—even those who take excellent steps toward good oral hygiene.

Many people think of elderly people as those who might be candidates for dental implants, but this is a misperception. People of all ages can be good candidates for this type of solution. People of every age might need dental work done on their teeth, dental implants or otherwise. Taking action sooner rather than waiting will lead to better health, and that is something to really smile about.

With tooth loss, regardless of the reason, with time comes loss of muscle mass and bone density in the face. This is a precursor to larger problems—problems that could be avoided with dental implants.

To show you just how diverse the group of people is that can benefit from dental implants, I want to share with you some brief examples of people who have come to my seminars and scheduled appointments with me at Custom Dental. Keep in mind, this is in Atoka County, Oklahoma, and a few surrounding areas, primarily, which has a sum total population of less than 20,000 people.

We've had the opportunity to help a young woman who was born with no front tooth. When she was seventeen, just preparing to start her adult life and determine what her career would be, she came in for a consultation so we could go over her options. She could have had a temporary partial that she'd take in and out, but that was sure to make her a target for other kids to tease and didn't really offer much more security than not having the tooth there. She didn't want that, her parents didn't want that, and we didn't want that for her. Another option was creating a bridge, but to do that you would have to cut into two perfectly good teeth to put it in, which is not ideal. The thought of intentionally damaging good teeth, especially to someone who is struggling with failing or missing teeth, is insane.

However, something had to be done, because when you do not have a tooth in an area, the bone has no reason to be there and it begins to melt away. The result is that you begin to experience bone loss. See Image (1) at the top of following page.

Image (1)

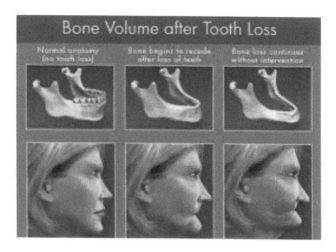

Once bone is gone, it's gone and bone loss still takes place with a bridge. What that meant to this young lady, in particular, was that by the time she turned thirty she would have to get the bridge redone because it would not fit well or look cosmetically pleasing. Then she'd have to do that same thing again at fifty. And then again, about every 10 to 20 years as life continued on, or until the anchor teeth ended up breaking because of the additional forces on them over the years. The big question: how could we avoid that?

Dental implants were the only permanent solution for this young lady. It would look great, fit her smile, and last forever. This is what she chose and from the day she received her implant, she was able to begin living her life with a higher level of confidence and less worry or self-scrutiny. Stories such as hers continue to motivate me and remind me that I am exactly where I'm meant to be, serving the people I'm meant to serve.

The most affordable and common dental practice is to simply pull a tooth to fix a problem.

Thankfully people don't tie a string to their tooth and attach something heavy to the end of it to extract teeth any longer—like the comedies and stories from long ago. They go to a dentist to get it pulled and they face the fact that they may not have that tooth any longer, but they don't have the pain either. Then that's it. They continue on through life minus that one tooth.

Many people simply do not realize that the loss of even a single tooth can compromise the mouth and create additional problems down the road.

By using a dental implant to replace even a single tooth, you will be healthier and feel better about yourself long term. Again, it's a permanent fix not a temporary patch job.

So many things can lead to poor oral health for us. Some are within our control and some are not in our control at all, but regardless of the "why", dental implants are often the solution. I'm always in an educate and inform mode, because my patients are owed that much with these big decisions, and I'm also just that passionate about how dental implants don't just change lives, they transform them.

The transformed smiles are the bonus at the end of the procedure!

I have the opportunity to host monthly seminars on dental implants. In these seminars we inform and educate the audience, and also have past patients come in to share their experiences. There is nothing more amazing than seeing someone who was not confident when you first met them go and talk about the confidence that their dental implants have given them. It's so inspiring!

Not so long ago, a past patient named Butch came in and allowed us to do a video testimonial of his experience. I wanted to share a bit of what he shared with all of us with you, because it really hits the nail on the head of people's mindsets when it comes to missing and failing teeth.

> *About ten years ago I lost my upper teeth. They came out due to chemo and a few other things that had happened years back. Everything had just taken its toll. I'd gotten partials and the experience was average at best, never really comfortable or efficient or really all that effective. And when you lose your teeth it's like losing your eyesight. You just cannot do the things you used to do.*
>
> *I'd always followed the "6-month rule", the one that says you can accept anything that happens to you after 6 months. Well, for me that meant that my partials were as good as I was going to get. Since they didn't work, I began to eat softer foods and not the right kinds of foods. I had to lose some weight in the end but I literally couldn't eat the foods that they were recommending. That's when I heard about Dr. Hookom and made an appointment. Today, I'm a healthier man and I try not to reflect on those experiences of the past, but I sure do enjoy the way I feel today. I have my life back and this outcome with the "6-month rule" is a heck of a lot better than the other one.* ~ Butch Pate

Every person we can reach and inform is a success in its own right, because we are letting them know that we understand, and more than that, we have solutions. Their concerns are valid and their desire for something more is valid, too. These people matter! That's why we work to:

- Help them learn about where they can turn to for reliable help
- Educate them in how to make smart choices regarding their oral health care
- Let them know that they do have an amazing smile that is ready to burst through
- Give solutions that will help to restore their confidence and allow them to begin to live life fully again—or maybe even for the first time

Many of the people we see already wear dentures. They have finally reached the point where they have to admit that they want better for themselves and more out of their lives. Our teeth are intricate to everything we do on a daily basis, including: eating, talking, and smiling. Dental implants offer solutions that help to alleviate:

- Loose, slipping dentures
- Electric shock pain that can occur when biting down
- Dealing with goopy, bad tasting adhesives
- Embarrassing clicking sounds while you speak or eat
- Impeded speech due to poor fit
- Continually reducing bone levels
- The assumption that you are older than you are; plus, you won't feel as old either
- The restrictions that affect the pleasure of eating

If you are a denture wearer, can you remember the last time you didn't have one or all of the concerns above? Do you like the thought of eliminating those concerns and tossing that denture case forever? If you think that sounds great, you'll want to consider dental implants further. Learn the basics, write down your questions, and seek out information for your specific situation.

Who cannot get dental implants?

There are only three absolute exceptions for people that disqualify them automatically from receiving dental implants. These are:
- Individuals who are pregnant
- Those who are HIV positive
- People who are suffering from uncontrolled diabetes

Are there other exceptions? Yes, there may be, but those can only be determined after a more thoughtful evaluation, one-on-one with a qualified professional in dental implants.

Find out if dental implants are a viable choice for you.

Amazing staff! They make you feel like you are a guest in their home. Dr. Hookom is extremely knowledgeable, friendly, and caring. I couldn't have asked for a better experience. They took great care of myself and my two daughters. We will be going back for dental work, and I look forward to it. It's not often you look forward to going to the dentist! ~ Kristina Milam, Atoka

CHAPTER 3

THE CONSIDERATIONS TO HELP DETERMINE IF DENTAL IMPLANTS ARE RIGHT FOR YOU

Sometimes your joy is the source of your smile, but sometimes your smile can be the source of your joy.
~ Thich Nhat Hanh

It is easy to understand how missing teeth can make someone feel less beautiful. They cover their mouth with their hand when they talk or smile; or worse, they look down because they feel embarrassed. Missing teeth are tough to deal with, and as a dentist, the concerns I have go beyond the person's smile, and right to their health.

Failing and missing teeth can cause many problems, including impacting the stability of the entire mouth, which results in:

- Gum (periodontal) disease
- Temporomandibular Joint (TMJ) symptoms
- Increased risk of diseases of the heart

These are challenging medical conditions for people which will wreak havoc on their quality of life. Dental implants are a solution that can help offer a higher quality of life, both physically and emotionally. This is why they are becoming a more sought out and viable option for people who need to address oral health concerns.

Below is Image (2), which shows us what physically happens to us when we lose our teeth:

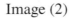

Image (2)

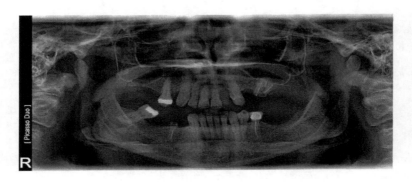

This image represents what bone loss and disease lead to. It impacts our bite, how we chew and swallow, and our sinus cavities also drop down when we do not have teeth in place due to the change from bone loss. Ultimately, this all leads to higher risk of cracking other teeth and additional tooth loss.

According to the American Academy of Implant Dentistry, research shows:
- More than 30 million Americans are missing all their teeth in one or both jaws
- 15 million people in the US have crown and bridge replacements for missing teeth
- 3 million have implants and that number is growing by 500,000 a year
- The success rate of dental implants has been reported in scientific literature as 98 percent
- The dental implant and prosthetic market in the US is projected to reach $6.4 billion by 2018

Dentist see implants as a viable option for restoring health. Customers in need of such services look to dental implants as a way to get back what broken, missing, or loose teeth have stolen from them.

Furthermore, according to Charles Mayo, co-founder of the esteemed Mayo Clinic: "People who keep their teeth live an average of ten years longer than people who lose their teeth due to poor nutrition." I think we can all agree that there is a lot of joy we can experience in our lives with up to an extra decade.

> *I had to have my first implant, yesterday. It was an older large filing by another dentist, and the filling and tooth broke as I was eating Christmas day. He thought he could save my tooth with a crown, but when he saw the tooth was cracked also, I had to have it pulled. I wasn't surprised, to find my tooth was cracked. Proud of my implant. So far, very little pain.* ~ Carolyn Robertson, Lane

Do I choose dentures, a bridge, or dental implants?

Dentures and bridges are considered more affordable options than dental implants and that is why so many people choose that route. However, unbeknownst to them many of the times, they do not understand the implications that current "affordability" can have on their long term wellbeing.

We can replace a single missing tooth or multiple missing teeth with dental implants. If you are having difficulty chewing or speaking because of missing teeth, dental implants may be the best solution for improving your quality of life. Many people may choose a single tooth denture because it is the most economical, but that will be in exchange for possible irritation, discomfort, replacement every 5 to 10 years, removal at night and continued bone loss.

To give you an idea, the image below (3) shows you a flipper denture:

Image (3)

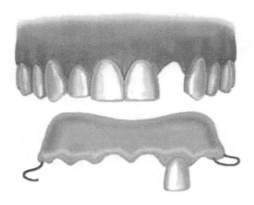

Another option is a Fixed Maryland Bridge, which is also fairly economical. The big downside to this is that you have to actually compromise two good teeth in order to get something that is semi-permanent. It will still have to be replaced every 5 to 10 years, as well, and the bone loss will continue. The image below (4) is what this option would look like:

Image (4)

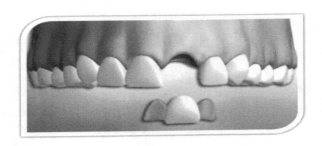

A step further, you can go with a Fixed Bridge, which is fixed and it is okay if adjoining teeth need crowns. However, you have to cut into healthy teeth to make this happen, which is risky, and it's easier for food to get trapped at the pontic. Plus, the bone loss continues! The image below (5) shows what this type of bridge looks like:

Image (5)

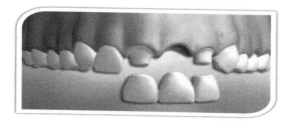

But...if you want permanent solutions that stop bone loss and other concerns that stem from that, you really do need to explore dental implants further to see if they are the right fit for you.

<u>With dental implants you can restore your smile.</u>
Many patients with missing teeth enjoy the benefits of being able to restore their smiles with dental implants. Your dental implant dentist will create a custom treatment plan to fill any gaps in your smile and restore optimal functioning of your mouth.

<u>Dental implants are a permanent tooth replacement solution.</u>
The downside to dental implants is that it is a costlier option initially than dentures or bridges, but the intangible benefits, as well as literal ones, make it hard to really place a price tag on that. In addition, it may take longer to complete the process, depending on the extent of the work, than it would take for dentures.

Here's an image (6) of what a dental implant looks like:

Image (6)

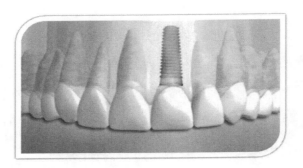

Dental implants and implant-supported dentures are a permanent tooth replacement solution for adults with missing teeth. There is no need for removable appliances, and the dental implant can help save the bone and surrounding tissue from deteriorating. Implants are a permanent solution for replacing missing teeth.

There are five (5) considerations that you should evaluate if you are beginning the process of determining if dental implants are the right option for you.

1. What is the quality of your life?

It can be hard to reconcile that the quality of our life in every way can be associated with our mouth and the condition of our teeth, but it is quite impactful. If you have missing teeth and put some thought into your life up to this point, do you...

- Recognize opportunities that you lost out on because you were too self- conscious to let yourself be known?
- Avoid pictures with loved ones who are smiling and happy because you do not want to smile?
- Not share your insights and thoughts because you don't want all eyes drawn to you?

Those are just three examples of how people who are insecure about missing teeth have struggles in their personal life. It's hard to forget the problem and it does take an emotional toll with many individuals.

If you have ever wondered what it would be like to…

- Smile with confidence at the people you love
- Eat your favorite foods without pain or embarrassment, or
- Feel 10 to 20 years younger

You need to consider dental implants. They offer you a whole new opportunity to live life on your terms, starting today.

2. Are you a good candidate?

At its basis, the need for dental implants stems from when you are missing some or all of the teeth in your arch. The arch is defined as the set of teeth that make up your lower or upper bite. And within the bite, you might be facing the loss of a single tooth only, which can likely be solved with a less intensive alternative. However, if you are missing several to all of your teeth, you will want to investigate more permanent solutions that will prevent further loss and decrease your chances of having the onset of additional health risks.

Please keep in mind, that implant dentistry isn't solely cosmetic in nature, although we understand the appeal of that. The reality is that from a functional perspective, missing teeth can create serious problems throughout the mouth and entire body. With even one missing tooth, bone loss begins and the shape of the mouth can actually shift—there's all this extra room for it to use. This all leads to a shift in the jaw, which eventually spreads throughout the body, leading to TMJ symptoms, which include:

- Dizziness

- Tinnitus (ringing of the ears)
- Headaches
- Soreness and stiffness in the neck, shoulders, and back

Four very uncomfortable and disruptive health problems, all stemming from the jaw shifting. So, yes, the sooner you address missing teeth, the better off you'll be.

Things get more challenging when you are missing all of your teeth. This is a tremendous loss emotionally, as well as in regards to the body's function. Over the decades, most people who have turned to dentures experience this and for some, dentures work great, but for many, dentures move and shift around, are hard to keep clean, and they don't look natural. Why is this? It's because you're only returning about 20% of function to your mouth with them. Dental Implants will take you to better results—80% or more! Better yet, these are permanent teeth that cannot be removed. They are a part of you, just like your original teeth were.

> *Dr. Hookom and staff were very professional, courteous, caring and knowledgeable. I appreciated their genuine and heartfelt concerns, it made my experience a blessing!! I'd highly recommend Custom Dental. Thank y'all.* ~ Shelly White, Atoka

3. Can you benefit from dental implants?

Our day to day lives are made more special by enjoying special moments with those we love or indulging in our favorite activities without fear or concern about what may happen as a result. Ask yourself this:

- Have you ever gone out to dine and didn't enjoy the meal, fearful of your dentures not cooperating?
- When is the last time you enjoyed your favorite food, such as an apple?

- Do you hesitate to talk at a natural level because of how your voice sounds?

If you have fears based on those three questions above, the benefits of dental implants may be more than what you may have thought possible. In fact, our patients have given us ten wonderful reasons why dental implants were the right choice for them. Perhaps you can relate to some of them, or at least a few.

#1: Appearance
Since dental implants look and feel like natural teeth, they help your mouth maintain a structure that those with their natural teeth would have. It's discreet and people notice your smile first and foremost.

#2: More opportunities for adventure
It's not easily recognizable until you're in the situation, but activities such as swimming, skiing, and even showing the dynamic side of you during a business presentation can be impacted when that voice in the back of your mind is reminding you that your dentures could slip at any moment.

#3: Mealtime
I've had patients who've confessed that they've never really enjoyed a meal when they've gone out to eat, moving the food around instead of daring to enjoy it—just in case. Dental implants give you the opportunity to truly participate in the meals you have with friends, families, and colleagues.

#4: Speech
Missing teeth or unreliable dentures affect the natural cadence and rhythm of your speech, creating a slight hissing sound or lisp-like intonation that can be distracting to you, as well as frustrating. This problem is alleviated with dental implants, as there is no risk of slipping. You have a story to tell and people want to hear it!

#5: Durability

Dental implants are durable, seldom needing to be replaced, regardless of the age when you get them. Taking good care of your implants is always the key to them lasting you a lifetime.

#6: Increase self-esteem

When we smile we feel better about ourselves. And when we feel better about ourselves our potential to make our lives as wonderful as possible skyrockets.

#7: Better oral health

Our teeth are necessary for many functions and for those who have healthy teeth remaining intact, dental implants do not require that you have to grind down on healthy teeth in order to fit dentures in. Furthermore, with individual implants, you can have better oral health between teeth to maintain healthier gums and implants.

#8: Less or eliminated discomfort

Because dental implants are permanent, the discomfort and soreness that comes from moving and loose dentures is virtually eliminated.

#9: Convenience

Not having to invest in messy pastes and cleaners to help keep your dentures clean and eliminate odor from them is very liberating. Most patients who choose dental implants find this freedom from concern to be wonderful. Brushing their teeth becomes that wonderful twice a day two-minute routine that others have.

#10: You deserve it

We often invest so much into others and their happiness, while not paying the proper attention to our needs and happiness. The people we love and care about want us to take care of ourselves, and permanent solutions to tough dental problems is something that is in your best interests health-wise and happiness-wise, which makes it a great choice for you.

4. Do you understand what dental implants are, exactly?

In the world of dentistry there have been incredible advancements over the years and things continue to get better. Dental implants have never been a greater choice for so many than they are today. Why? Because the implants look and perform like our natural teeth would, as they are rooted into the bone there is no artificial plastic on the roof of the mouth or the need to have adhesives and creams in order for the teeth to be functional.

As a professional in dental implants, the one benefit I find to be exceptional is that when you have dental implants, you're not asking adjacent teeth to carry the load, which means there is less stress on them and therefore, the risk of healthy teeth becoming compromised is reduced.

The dental implant becomes the long-lasting tooth root and it is fastened right into the jaw bone, which gives it the look, feel, and function of a natural tooth. There's no movement or shifting.

There are three parts to the dental implants that are available today. They are:

The titanium implant

This is fused directly to the jawbone. Titanium is used because it is easily accepted by the body and the bone grows around the specially-designed titanium implant in a process called osseointegration.

The abutment

This part of the Dental Implant fits over the portion of the implant that protrudes from the gum line.

The crown

This is the tooth that becomes a part of your new permanent set of teeth.

Below is an image (7) that gives a side by side comparison of the natural tooth to the dental implant:

Image (7)

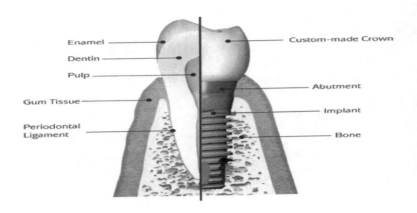

Enamel — Custom-made Crown

Dentin —

Pulp —

— Abutment

Gum Tissue —

— Implant

Periodontal
Ligament — Bone

5. How would your life have changed if you considered implants sooner?

When you reflect on the lost opportunities in your life—moments of joy and things you wanted to do but were too leery to attempt because you lacked the confidence, it's easy to see how dental implants could have given you more chances to embrace your life more. Today is the day that you need to think about and what it is you want from this moment forward. If you don't want to be held back due to failing teeth, you are never too old or young to consider dental implants. Your happiness does matter, and there is nothing that brings me greater joy than seeing the smile return to my patients' faces after they see themselves with their implants for the first time.

A powerful story...

All our patients are important to us, but occasionally we meet someone whose story is so touching and challenging that it really leaves an impact and gives us a reminder of what we all truly have to be grateful for in our lives.

A veteran came in to see me who'd lost some limbs and appendages. It had been some time ago and over the years his teeth had really deteriorated, to the point where there were only a few left and those that remained were broken and infected. One option for him was dentures—not ideal, but an option. There was also the choice of snap-in dentures, see figure (8), but with his disabilities and the loss of some limbs grabbing the denture to insert it and take it out would have been very difficult for him so it really wasn't a feasible choice, as he couldn't physically do it.

Image (8)

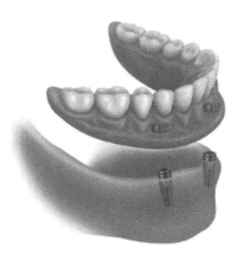

After discussing what implants could do to help him today to make his life better and healthier, he chose an option called our perma-bridge. This is the best option for someone that is missing most or all of their teeth. This is the Cadillac of dentistry. See Figure (9).

Image (9)

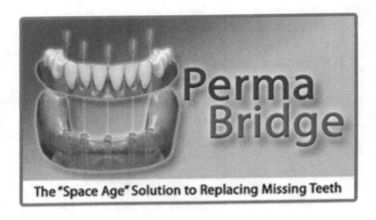

A perma-bridge is where the dentist places 4 to 6 implants on top and on bottom arch and place porcelain crowns permanently on those implants. Yes, I said permanently. They never come off. This technology is like having all their own teeth again! This option was something that would work perfectly for him with his limited function, but it was also something that gave him hope and a smile! Today, our well deserving veteran is a happier and healthier man and his situation is just a bit easier. The blessed feeling that comes from knowing that we were able to help in a compassionate and professional way are incredible.

Visiting Custom Dental was truly unlike any dental experience I have ever had. The workplace was fun (I know that's almost unbelievable for a dental experience), patient-centered, productive, and all staff members were interested in meeting the needs of the patient. Emily became my "best friend" in her care for me, and Dr. Hookom was the best! A "no pain" experience. A very big difference maker...one appointment gave me a comprehensive exam as a new patient, cleaning, and preparation for a cracked tooth. From my previous experiences with dental offices, that would have been three separate visits with wait time in between. Congratulations, Custom Dental, a new management style that outshines them all!
~ Anonymous

CHAPTER 4

THE "MUST–KNOWS" ABOUT DENTAL IMPLANTS

A warm smile is the universal language of kindness.
~ William Arthur Ward

As a dentist who specializes in dental implants, I have great insight to offer clients into everything that they must know in order to make the impactful choices in their life regarding the implant procedure and decision. Occasionally, there will be patients who may need to be referred over to an oral surgeon and in those cases, the referral is definitely made and recommended. However, through consultations with possible dental implant recipients, we go through a thorough history and examination to help us come to the solutions that will change their lives in an exciting way.

The Big Question...

Does it hurt? Everyone asks this and we don't blame them! It is less uncomfortable and painful than what you may imagine. Through the use of a local anesthesia there is minimal discomfort during the procedure. Most patients report only minimal post-op discomfort and can return to work the next day, using nothing more than an over-the-counter medication such as Advil or Tylenol to feel comfortable. Plus, by following the proper post-op instructions for care, you will find that your healing process is one that you can manage, even be excited about, because such an exciting new phase to your life is about to begin.

> *Dr. Hookom and his staff are a top notch team. They are all excellent at what they do and the atmosphere is very friendly and professional. I would recommend them to anyone looking for a great dental experience.*
> ~ Barry Nesterud, Marietta

Here are some interesting facts about missing teeth and tooth loss:

- Many older adults end up losing all of their natural teeth
- Almost 180 million people in the US are missing at least one tooth
- Approximately 4 percent of adults do not have any teeth
- Diet and nutrition play an important role in maintaining your teeth

These numbers are staggering and they are why I will at least recommend listening to the options and reasons why dental implants may be the best solution for a patient. It's a productive and informational conversation, never a pressure salesman approach. My staff and I truly want what's best for our patients and potential patients, alike. Science, technology, and results indicate that dental implants have to be a part of that conversation.

We share the specifics on why implant supported dentures work. You see, they are designed to rely on a set of dental implants that attach to the base of custom dentures. These dentures provide more of a secure fit than traditional dentures. The most popular kind of implant denture we do is called our snap-in denture. This procedure ensures a secure fit and the elimination of the need for messy denture pastes and creams.

With Locator Overdenture Implant System (LODI), or as we call it our snap-in denture, which was Image (8). We have found it to be an ideal solution for many of our patients who have lost all or most of their teeth and who may have severe bone loss in the jaw. Typically, patients with severe bone loss would require bone grafting procedures to ensure that there is enough bone for the implant to integrate with. However, with LODI system, patients can skip these additional surgeries and have their implant supported denture placed almost immediately. The LODI system, Image (8), is noninvasive, predictable, and durable dental implant option.

Effective, strategic, and compassionate consultations

There are five unique elements to the consultations that I have with people regarding dental implants. I feel that each of these is very important to address, whether someone is meeting with me at Custom Dental or with another dental implant provider. This is one of the biggest decisions that many people will make in their lives and the more informed they are, the better our experience together is. And the reality is that the longer you wait to make these important decisions, the more at risk you become to further problems and concerns. As with all things regarding our health and wellbeing that are not attended to in a timely manner—they often become worse. Don't wait until it may be too late.

1. **The reasons that dental implants may not be a good choice for you.**
   We all have a different health history and set of circumstances in our lives that dictate whether certain procedures are recommended for us or not. Through the specific training regarding dental implants that I have received, we go through a thorough check to make sure that the implants are indeed the best choice for you. A few things that you can expect to have us cover is:

   - Allergies and known adverse reactions to medications and local anesthetics that may be part of the procedure
   - Complete medical history
   - All oral health and wellbeing concerns

While having concerns about any of the items listed above isn't an automatic disqualifier, it can play a role in how we approach both your procedure and the recovery time after it is complete. The more information we have the better. Your best outcome is always the primary goal.

2. The training that the dentist has received.

My commitment to continuing, extensive education and certification in dental implants and technology is a core part of my commitment to my clients and my commitment to serving them at the highest level of excellence possible. The best technology in the world when it comes to dental implants is the Cone Beam 3d x-ray machine. This technology allows your dentist to see the width, length, and density of the bone. See Image (10) below.

Image (10)

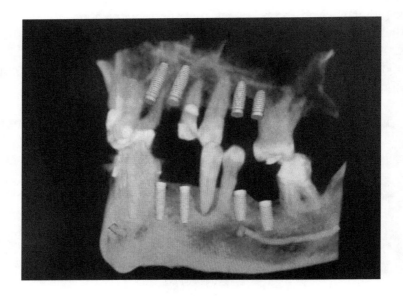

The Cone Beam machine also allows me to see the location of all the nerves and sinuses. Make sure your implant dentist has this technology before you say yes to your dental implant.

In addition to my commitment, everyone who works with my patients has that same goal. It's our efforts as a team that give you the smile you've been longing to get back, or find for the first time. Whether you are visiting with my staff and I at Custom Dental or another provider of implants, please make sure that you are not hesitant to ask any and all questions that are important. Whoever is talking with you should be glad to share as much information as possible with you to help alleviate your concerns and calm your fears or nerves. In addition, they should have the expertise and insight to lay out the scenarios for you, and guide you through what the entire process will be from start to finish.

3. The success rate of the dental implants performed.

As referenced earlier, the success rate of dental implants is quite high. As a reminder, according to the AAID, the success rate is estimated at 98% still after 10 years, according to research and reported results. This is one of the highest success rates you will find out of any procedure, medical or cosmetic.

When it comes to the specific dentist that you choose to work with for your implants, there should be referrals available where past patients share their outcomes and experience with you. We celebrate our referrals, as they are successes and post them in video testimonies, as well as on our website, and yes, even in this book. Your level of comfort with us means everything to us and we will go out of our way with sincere efforts and desires to show you that we take care of you as if you are a member of our family. And after our time together, you truly do become a part of our family.

4. Understanding what would make a dental implant rejection.

While odds of success and the proven history of dental implants are definitely in your favor, the noted reasons that a rejection could occur include:

- Contamination
- Infection
- Too much pressure during placement
- Too much moving during healing phase
- Patient's oral hygiene habits
- 5 to 10% of failures are due to unknown factors
- Smoking interferes with healing and can reduce success rate

5. A thorough understanding of your entire procedure.

One wonderful thing about dental implants is that the process is easy to define for patients so they can anticipate exactly what is going to happen. All situations that may create a variance can be spoken of in general terms prior to the procedure, but as a standard, they seldom become reality. Through your understanding of what to expect during a procedure (as most procedures can cause anxiety), we will work together to:

- Lessen anxiety, through a combination of sedation dentistry, a wonderful "chair-side manner", and keeping you informed in a calm and nurturing way. It is only in very rare circumstances that you would ever require more than a local anesthesia.
- Let you know what the expectations will be for follow-up and post procedure care.
- Show you the compassion that you deserve and want during this exciting opportunity to make a significant, positive impact in your life.
- Inform you. Actual implant placement takes approximately 30 to 60 minutes per implant. A full

case completion may take from 3 weeks to 9 months depending on treatment plan, bone quality, and the number of implants placed.
- Alleviate worries—you are never without teeth!
- Go through a thorough analysis of all cost and fees associated with the procedure, based on your specific scenario, along with financing options to help you if your insurance does not cover this type of procedure (which few dental plans do, as they focus on prevention mostly).

You've learned some great information and I'm very excited that you've allowed me to share it with you. Through requesting this book, you've shown how serious you are about making some big changes in your life that will help guide you toward better health, a happier perspective, and a genuine smile that starts from the inside and works its way out.

> *I am a faithful client, for I believe in total health accountability and that includes dental health. The facility, staff, and precious Dr. Hookom presents the best care for my dental health and me as a person. I think the staff secretly researches (ha!) your life and interests because when you walk in and talk, they seem to actually "know" you. No hype, no pressured sales of products, just care and honesty. PS: I love the music also. I literally have to contain myself...I could just go there daily for a little R and R!* ~ Kathy Perkins, Atoka

CHAPTER 5

YOU'RE READY TO START. WHAT'S NEXT?

Here's wishing you the smiles o' life and not a single grumble.
~ Irish Blessing

People with dental implants tell us they feel better, look better, and live better. It's a life changing experience for them and we get to contribute to that! That is the pinnacle of success and the evidence that we're all working with our gifts in a passionate and professional manner.

The joy that comes from seeing people once again talk, laugh, and eat comfortably with family, friends, and co-workers, without being hostage to their teeth is amazing. And the common thing we hear every patient say when they are done is, "I wish I had done this sooner."

You don't need to wait, and we are here to help. I'm proud to be known as "Your Atoka Dentist", because I do love being your dentist. My team and I strive to create a relationship with you that lets you know that you are appreciated as a person, not just as a patient.

Our practice is modern and state of the art, because with all of the amazing services we offer, even aside from dental implants, we want to give people the best. When someone walks into Custom

Dental, long gone are the days of those "tough dentist stories." We don't operate that way. We work with people to walk them through their fears and to a better place. This is an intangible part of our business that could never have a price. Our patients know we are always there for them.

> *I was so afraid to even go to a Dentist, but knew I needed to. Two of my good friends, Becky and Polly recommended Dr. Hookom, I'm so glad they did.*
>
> *I called and set up an appointment, No Insurance mind you. Dr. Hookom took me in and x-rayed and counseled me on the work I needed done and told me how much it would cost and made me a plan that I could afford.*
>
> *The hidden costs were NONE. I was so pleased with all the Ladies from the front desk to the Dentist Chair, they are so sweet and kind. Being the Big Chicken I am, I felt very at ease and cared for. I will continue to go there because it was a joy, and the work done was of excellent quality and looked great!!!* ~ Leda Canida, Colgate

Our commitment to excellence means that you can benefit from working with an experienced, professional, and knowledgeable team of dental professionals. We are masters of the smile and bringing out the best smile you have is something we are proud of. There are few testaments more powerful than someone leaving a dentist office smiling and happy, then sharing that smile with everyone around them and maybe even their story.

Giving of our gifts and giving back

Our entire team is dedicated to serving the community and helping others. We believe and know that by showing God's love and serving through our practice, we can do great things for many people. This is why we have a program called Free Dental Day, where we offer fillings, extractions, and cleanings absolutely free. We do this once and sometimes twice a year to thank and serve our community. I also participate in school education programs and do free visual exams. We love serving our community, and would love for you to be a part of our family!

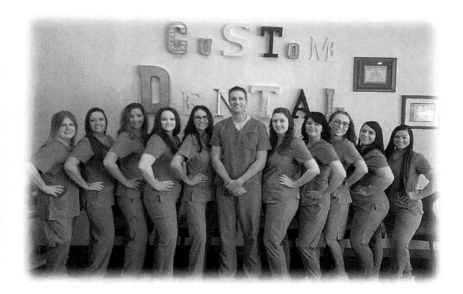

Taking care of our family

Since we are community minded, we treat everyone that walks through our door like our family. And what do we do with family? We take care of them, and are there for them when they need us. While we perform many procedures for our patients that transform their lives, the work we do through dental implants continues to inspire all of us. I always smile when I hear people mention that they're surprised that such a high level of dental care exists right in little Atoka. Well, Atoka maybe small in population, but it's big in heart, spirit to help, and excellence. That's what our office Custom Dental is all about; we pride ourselves in knowing everyone's name and caring about their lives, not just their business. I think that's what makes us so special. Because every smile has a story and every person can have a smile!

When people walk in to visit us for dental implants, they are usually nervous and a bit self-conscious. It's awkward to talk about something that is so personal and they are often resistant to get their hopes up too high. There is much to learn and a lot they need to know. On your first visit with us at Custom Dental, this is what you can expect:

- A comprehensive exam with me
- To receive digital x-rays so we can see a clear image of what is happening with your teeth and the overall state of your oral health
- To do a complete health history together so we can help determine any factors that may be of concern
- A detailed custom treatment plan that would work for you, including a breakdown of the exact recommended procedures and costs

Your first appointment usually takes about an hour to go through everything, but depending on your questions and concerns and what needs to be done to give you a thorough picture of what your process might be and what you can expect, it can take longer. We take the time to make sure we're addressing all of your needs and don't want to cut you short. This is important, and we get that!

During the consultation with me, you have a perfect opportunity to ask as many questions as you may have about procedures and oral health, in general. The more information you leave our office with, the better equipped you will be to determine the right course of action for you.

I love the staff!!! Before coming to Custom Dental I was death grip afraid of dental offices. Chalk it up to a really bad experience in my childhood, but I literally wouldn't go for cleanings or pain.

After going to Dr. Hookom, I am no longer scared, I go every six months like clockwork and have even opted for some intense dental repair. I couldn't be happier!
~ Deann Jackson, Coalgate

"Get your smile and get your life back!"

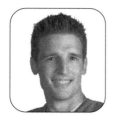

About Dr. Matt Hookom, DDS

Since 2009, Dr. Matthew Hookom has been practicing advanced preventative and restorative dentistry in the Atoka, Oklahoma, serving the community and surrounding areas. His passion for helping give people the confidence to smile shows through in his work and he continually strives to help his patients achieve excellent oral health care through exceptional care and personalized patient education. This is an important mission for him in his daily work, because problems of the mouth often lead to health problems in other parts of the body.

The Doctor's mission to bring back one smile at a time to his clients is a driving force in his life. Dr. Hookom says, "Each patient comes in with their own concerns. It is up to me to help them understand the risks of not taking action, while showing them what they can do to promote healthy teeth and gums." His practice, Custom Dental of Atoka, offers services which include: Dental Implants; Cosmetic Dentistry; Orthodontics, Laser Gum Therapy; Smile Makeover; Periodontal Care; and, All-On-4 Implant Supported Dentures.

Dr. Hookom received his Doctor of Dental Surgery (DDS) degree from the University of Oklahoma Health Science Center. He is a member of the American Dental Association, the Oklahoma Dental Association, the Academy of General Dentistry, and the American Orthodontic Association. In the rapidly advancing world of Dentistry, he is committed to staying abreast of new trends in dental care and cutting-edge technology. He also continues to pursue extensive post-doctoral training, which specifically includes: oral conscious sedation; implantology, orthodontics, endodontics, and cosmetic dentistry.

One of the greatest joys in Dr. Hookom's personal life is to spend time with his wife Emily and their two wonderful children, Belle and Luke. Together, they enjoy hunting and fishing. Any opportunity to be outdoors and a bit closer to nature is something that brings them all a smile.

Contact Us

We encourage you to reach out to us.
If you have questions, we can help you find the answers.
www.atokadentist.com

Custom Dental
1828 W. Liberty Road
Atoka, OK 74525

New Patients Number: 580-889-7788
Current Patients Number: 580-889-7900

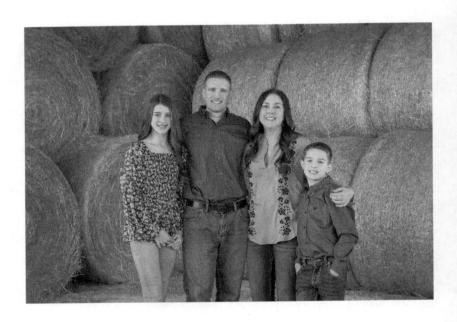